THE DUKAN DIET FOR ATHLETES

A Culinary Journey to Health and Vitality

Parker Jones

Table of Contents:

Introduction

In New York City, where life goes quickly, Andrew was seen as the most energetic and athletic person of his time. He pushed himself to the edge in the gym and on the field when he was young. He lived for the thrill of the game. But Andrew found that he was having weight problems, even though he loved sports. His love of sugary snacks and fast food seemed to get in the way of his hard workout routine, leaving him tired and unhappy with his body.

In order to get his energy back and do his best, Andrew started the Dukan Diet, which would change his life forever. Andrew was hesitant at first after meeting a close friend who had read my book and done very well on the diet plans I suggested. But he couldn't deny that his friend's look and energy levels had changed clearly.

Andrew was excited to try the Dukan Diet because it focused on veggies, lean meats, and healthy ways of living. An overflow of tasty and filling foods caught his attention, making him want to move around and eat more. Delicious chicken skewers and rich cottage cheese pancakes were among the delectable meals that became symbols of his commitment to life and health.

As the weeks went by, Andrew's hard work paid off. The weight disappeared, showing a stronger, slimmer body underneath. But Andrew's appearance was not the only thing that changed; his general state of health also saw a big alteration. His confidence shot through the roof, his energy levels soared, and he developed a fresh, renewed love for the game.

Andrew is excited to share his journey with others now that he has hit the peak of his sporting ability. He offers a call to you to begin your own culinary adventure toward health and vigor with the Dukan Diet through the pages of this cookbook. The recipes and insights found in these pages provide a route to success for anyone wanting to lose weight and feel better, or for the more experienced athlete trying to maximize performance.

Join Andrew and numerous others who have chosen the Dukan Diet as a way of life that supports wellness and vitality rather than just helping people lose weight. Use this cookbook as a roadmap to help you on your path to a

better, happy you as you learn about
the transformational power of healthy,
delectable food.

Chapter One

Understanding the Dukan Diet

We cover the basic ideas of the Dukan Diet in this foundational chapter to give you a full grasp of this well-known weight loss plan. This part is your indispensable guide to getting the benefits of this life-changing program, regardless of your level of experience with the Dukan Diet.

The Principles of the Dukan Diet: Attack, Cruise, Consolidation, and Stabilization arc thc four key steps of the diet that we will first review. Every stage has been carefully planned to maximize weight loss, encourage wholesome living, and ensure long-term success. You'll learn the reasons behind each stage and how it helps with long-term weight control, from the protein-rich Attack Phase to the Consolidation Phase's slow return of some foods.

Benefits of the Dukan Diet: Next, we'll review the Dukan Diet's numerous advantages that go beyond just helping people lose weight. The benefits of the Dukan Diet go well beyond weight loss; they include lower hunger, better digestion, more energy, and improved mental focus. Based on empirical studies and personal anecdotes, we examine the comprehensive benefits of this well-known program and its potential to completely change your wellness and health practice.

Getting Started: Step-by-Step Guide: Lastly, we show you a full road map so you may start your Dukan Diet journey with clarity and confidence. With this detailed guide, you will learn how to determine your True Weight and build a customized food plan, giving you the tools and information that you need to be successful right now. We're here to help you every step of the way, whether you're making your first Dukan-friendly meal or navigating the grocery store aisles.

You will have a full idea of the Dukan Diet's principles, advantages, and workable application methods by the end of this chapter. Equipped with this understanding, you'll be prepared to bravely and happily set out on a transforming culinary adventure towards health and vitality.

The Principles of the Dukan Diet
The Dukan Diet runs on a set of rules that stress the consumption of lean protein, support moderate weight loss, and support long-term weight maintenance. To properly follow the Dukan Diet and meet your wellness and health goals, it is important to understand these principles. Here is a full examination of the main thoughts behind the Dukan Diet:

1. Protein as the Foundation: The Dukan Diet puts a strong focus on lean protein as the main source of nutrients. The main component of every meal is protein, which may be found in chicken, fish, lean meats, eggs, and low-fat dairy goods. Protein helps you feel fuller for longer periods of time and lessens cravings for bad snacks. It is also important for the growth and repair of cells.

2. Four Unique stages: The Dukan Diet is broken down into four unique stages, each of which has a different role in the process of losing weight:

- Attack Phase: Usually lasting two to seven days, this initial phase exclusively focuses on foods high in protein to improve weight loss.

- Cruise Phase: During this stage, lean proteins and non-starchy veggies are gradually reintroduced to promote continued weight loss until the goal weight is met.

- Consolidation Phase: This phase gradually adds more meals while sticking to the diet's rules to stop rebound weight gain.

- Stabilization Phase: This last stage concentrates on maintaining weight loss through the adoption of wholesome eating habits and regular exercise.

3. No Calorie Counting: This diet makes calorie counting easier by emphasizing food quality over amount, in opposition to many fad diets that demand exact calorie counts. Protein-rich foods are chosen, and in later stages, the diet includes plenty of fruits, vegetables, and whole grains, which automatically controls calorie intake without the need for rigorous calorie management.

4. Emphasis on Water and Physical Exercise: Two important parts of the Dukan Diet are regular physical exercise and good hydration. Getting enough water improves digestion, encourages happiness, and helps in the removal of toxins from the body. In a similar way, adding regular

exercise not only helps with weight loss but also boosts general health and wellbeing.

5. Personalized Approach: The Dukan Diet acknowledges that every person is different and has various dietary needs, preferences, and goals. It therefore supports a customized approach to meal planning and diet modification to fit unique lives and nutritional decisions.

Followers of the Dukan Diet can build lasting habits for vitality and wellbeing, achieve sustained weight loss, and improve general health by following to these core principles.

Benefits of the Dukan Diet

The Dukan Diet is a holistic strategy to getting general health and well-being since it gives numerous benefits beyond just weight loss. People who follow its food standards and stick to its principles can reap a host of benefits that go well beyond the numbers on the scale. The following are the major benefits of the Dukan diet:

1. Effective Weight Loss: One of the Dukan Diet's most important perks is how well it works to promote weight loss. The diet supports quick initial weight loss during the Attack Phase, followed by steady and long-lasting weight loss over the following phases by stressing the consumption of lean protein and avoiding processed carbohydrates and sugars. This lowers the chance of obesity-related health problems while also helping people in reaching their goal weight.

2. Better Metabolic Health: The Dukan Diet has a strong focus on reducing blood sugar levels and improving metabolic processes, which can improve glucose metabolism and insulin sensitivity. Less consumption of high-glycemic carbs and a focus on lean foods and veggies high in fiber helps to lower insulin resistance, normalize blood sugar levels, and improve metabolic health in general.

3. Increased Energy: The diet prioritizes nutrient-dense foods that easily fuel the body, providing a constant source of energy in contrast to crash diets that frequently leave people feeling tired and lethargic. Meals high in protein can help control blood sugar levels and give you steady energy throughout the day, which can boost your energy, mental focus, and general efficiency.

4. Less Hunger and wants: Protein is well-known for its satiating qualities, which help people feel fuller for longer amounts of time and lessen desires for sugary and unhealthy snacks. The Dukan Diet helps lower hunger and cravings by including enough lean protein in each meal, which makes it easier to follow the plan and avoid temptation.

5. Preservation of Lean Muscle Mass: The Dukan Diet puts a high focus on keeping lean muscle mass, in opposition to many crash diets that cause both fat and muscle loss. The diet helps people lose extra body fat while keeping muscle power by giving enough protein and including strength training activities. This helps functional exercise and long-term

metabolic health in addition to better physical beauty.

6. Support for Cardiovascular Health: Lean meats, fish, nuts, seeds, and olive oil are heart-healthy foods high in vitamins, omega-3 fatty acids, and other nutrients important to cardiovascular health. These foods are also stressed in the Dukan Diet. A diet high in heart-healthy elements and low in processed foods and saturated fats can help lower the chance of heart disease and improve cardiac health in general.

7. Sustainable Lifestyle Changes: The Dukan Diet gives a sustainable approach to good food and lifestyle choices, in opposition to many fad diets that are hard to stick to in the long run. The diet aids people in building enduring habits that support

long-term health and wellbeing by gently reintroducing foods in later phases and giving directions for keeping a healthy weight for the rest of their lives.

All things considered, the Dukan Diet offers a thorough approach to weight loss and general health, giving people the tools and resources they require to reach their goals and lead full, busy lives. The Dukan Diet can be an effective tool in your desire for a healthy, happy you, whether your goals are to lose extra weight, gain better digestive health, or improve your general well-being.

Getting Started: Step-by-Step Guide

Starting the Dukan Diet is an exciting and life-changing way to reach your health and exercise goals. You can start the Dukan Diet with ease and confidence if you read this full guide. It has all the knowledge and tools you need.

1. Calculate Your True Weight:

The first step of the Dukan Diet is to find your True Weight, which is the weight that a healthy life will keep off on its own. This personalized calculator sets a fair and attainable weight loss goal by taking into account things like age, height, gender, and body composition.

2. Understand the four stages:

Learn about the four different phases of the Dukan Diet: Attack, Cruise, Consolidation, and Stabilization.

This process of losing weight has different steps, each with its own rules and things that are allowed. If you know why each step is important and how long it takes, you can use the tool better and get better results.

3. Stock Up on Dukan-Friendly Foods.

Check your freezer, fridge, and store to see what things are Dukan-friendly and follow the diet's rules. This includes non-starchy veggies, eggs, tofu, and lean proteins like chicken, turkey, fish, lean beef cuts, and low-fat dairy products. Keeping these wholesome basics on hand will ease the process of planning and cooking meals.

4. Plan Your Meals:

Following the Dukan Diet properly needs careful meal planning. Make sure that every meal has a mix of veggies, healthy fats, and lean protein when you plan your meals and snacks for the upcoming week. To keep your meals interesting and satisfying, try out several recipes and taste combos.

5. Drink Enough Water:

Maintaining proper hydration is important for supporting weight loss and general wellness. Drink eight glasses of water or more a day, and to please your taste without consuming more sugar or calories, try blending herbal teas, infused water, and sparkling water.

6. Include Regular Exercise:

Although the Dukan Diet mainly focuses on dietary changes, including regular exercise can improve weight reduction results and advance general health and well-being. Whether it's walking, running, riding, swimming, or strength training, choose something you want to do and try to get in at least 30 minutes of exercise most days of the week.

7. Monitor Your Progress: Throughout the Dukan Diet, keep an eye on your weight, measures, and general physical and mental well-being to chart your progress. Celebrate your success along the journey, whether it's hitting a large weight reduction milestone, downsizing to a lower size, or feeling an increase in general well-being and vitality.

You'll be well on your way to reaching your health and wellness goals and living a lively, energetic life if you adhere to the Dukan Diet's rules and follow these guidelines. Keep in mind that persistence, patience, and consistency are important, and view the journey as a chance for personal growth.

Chapter Two

Attack Phase Recipes

The Dukan Diet's Attack Phase is meant to help you lose weight quickly by emphasizing foods that are high in protein and low in carbohydrates. You will mostly eat lean proteins throughout this period to speed up fat burning and boost your metabolism. These meals from the Attack Phase are not only tasty but also nourishing, giving you the drive and contentment that you require to be successful in your weight loss efforts.

Components:

One pound (450 grams) of chunked, skinless, deboned, chicken breasts

1 tbsp of olive oil

One tbsp of paprika

Half a tsp of chili powder

½ tsp of powdered garlic

Add salt and pepper to savor

Guidelines:

To prepare a marinade, add the olive oil, paprika, cayenne pepper, garlic powder, salt, and pepper in a saucer.

Toss to coat the chicken chunks evenly after adding them to the marinade. Cover it and chill for at least 30 minutes.

Increase the heat to medium-high on the grill or grill pan. The marinated chicken portions are pierced onto skewers.

The chicken skewers should be cooked through and gently browned after 6 to 8 minutes of grilling on each side.

Enjoy while hot!

40 minutes for preparation

Smoked Salmon Roll-Ups:

Components:

Four oz (115g) portions of smoked salmon

Four ounces (115 grams) of cream cheese with less fat

1 tbsp of freshly sliced dill

1 tbsp of optional capers

Guidelines:

Mix the sliced fresh dill and low-fat cream cheese in a small saucer and stir until they mix properly.

Arrange the pieces of smoked salmon on a sanitized surface. Cover each slice uniformly using a slim layer of the cream cheese blend.

Sprinkle capers over the cream cheese blend if desired.

Form each piece of smoked salmon into a roll-up by tightly rolling it up.

Cut the roll-ups into bite-sized pieces, and if desired, use toothpicks to hold them in place.

Serve as a tasty, high-protein snack or starter.

Ten minutes for preparation

Components:

One pound (450 grams) of big de-skinned and deveined shrimp

2 chopped cloves of garlic

1 lemon's juice and zest

1 tbsp of olive oil

Add salt and pepper to improve its flavor

Decorate it with freshly chopped parsley

Guidelines:

To prepare a marinade, put the chopped garlic, olive oil, lemon zest, lemon juice, salt, and pepper in a basin.

Join the de-skinned and deveined shrimp with the marinade and toss until coated evenly. Cover and keep in the refrigerator for a quarter to half an hour.

In a frying pan, preheat the heat to medium-high. As the shrimp turn pink and opaque, add the marinated shrimp to the frying pan and cook for two to three minutes on each side.

As a decoration, scatter freshly cut parsley atop the cooked shrimp.

Serve hot with a crisp green salad or a side of steaming veggies.

20 minutes to half an hour for preparation

Tofu Stir-Fry:

Components:

Four hundred grams, or fourteen ounces of extra-firm, pressed, drained tofu

Two teaspoons of soy sauce (you can use tamari if you're gluten-free)

One tsp rice vinegar

One tsp of sesame oil

1 tbsp of olive oil

2 chopped garlic cloves

1 tbsp of nicely minced ginger

1 bell pepper, cut finely

1 cup florets of broccoli

1 cup of chopped mushrooms

Add salt and pepper to relish

Sliced green onions for the decoration

Guidelines:

Slice the compressed tofu into small cubes.

To prepare the sauce, mix the sesame oil, rice vinegar, and soy sauce in a little saucer.

In a big frying pan or wok, warm the olive oil over medium-high heat. Cook the grated ginger and chopped garlic for a minute, or until fragrant.

When the tofu cubes are golden brown on all sides, which should take five to seven minutes, add them to the frying pan.

Cook the broccoli florets, chopped mushrooms, and chopped bell pepper in the frying pan for a further five minutes, or until the veggies are a bit soft.

Sprinkle the tofu and veggies with the sauce, then mix to ensure even coating. Cook until well cooked, 2 to 3 minutes more.

Before serving, add salt and pepper to taste and garnish with sliced green onions.

Thirty minutes for preparation

Turkey Meatballs:

Components:

1 pound (450g) of lean ground turkey

¼ cup oat bran

1egg

Two sliced garlic cloves

1 tsp of dehydrated oregano

1 tsp of dried basil

Half a tsp of powdered onion

To taste, add salt and pepper.

Cook with olive oil.

Guidelines:

Lean ground turkey, oat bran, egg, minced garlic, dried oregano, dried basil, onion powder, salt, and pepper should all be mixed in a big blending basin.

After thoroughly mixing, form the blend into little meatballs.

In a frying pan over medium heat, warm the olive oil. When the meatballs are browned and well cooked, add them to the frying pan and cook for 6 to 8 minutes, turning them over once or twice.

For a satisfying supper, serve hot with your preferred Dukan-friendly sauce or with steamed veggies.

Twenty minutes for preparation

Chapter Three

Cruise Phase Recipes

You will continue to emphasize lean proteins as you move from the Dukan Diet's Attack Phase to its Cruise Phase, progressively adding non-starchy veggies back into your meals. With a greater range of food alternatives available during this phase, you can still support your weight loss objectives while increasing your culinary inventiveness. These tasty and nourishing Cruise Phase dishes will keep you moving in the direction of reaching your desired weight and enhancing your general health.

Grilled Turkey Breast With Herbs:

Components:

- Two tsp of olive oil

- Four turkey breast fillets

- Two mashed garlic cloves

- Lemon wedges for serving

- 1 tbsp each of minced fresh rosemary and thyme

- Salt & pepper to relish

Guidelines:

1. To prepare a marinade, add olive oil, mashed garlic, minced thyme, sliced rosemary, and salt and pepper in a little saucer.

2. Move the turkey breast fillets to a shallow plate and mask them with marinade, ensuring that they are coated completely. Cover it and chill for a minimum of half an hour.

3. Set the grill's temperature to medium-high. Take out the marinated turkey breast fillets and throw away any extra marinade.

4. Simmer the turkey breast fillets until the juices dry up and they are cooked through, 6 to 8 minutes on each side.

5. For a refreshing taste, serve hot with lemon slices on the side.

Set Up Time: thirty minutes

Zucchini Noodles With Pesto:

Components:

- Four medium zucchini

- A quarter cup of pine nuts

- One cup of fresh basil leaves

- Two garlic cloves

- A quarter cup of olive oil

- A quarter cup of shredded Parmesan cheese

- Spice with salt and pepper

- Decorate with cherry tomatoes (noncompulsory)

Guidelines:

1. Spiralize or use a vegetable peeler to make zucchini noodles, then separate them.

2. Put the parmesan cheese, pine nuts, garlic, olive oil, salt, and pepper in a food processor together with the basil leaves. To achieve the needed consistency, add additional olive oil if necessary, after pulsing until smooth and fully mixed.

3. Raise the temp to medium in a frying pan. When the zucchini noodles are warmed up but still crisp, put them in the frying pan and cook for two to three minutes.

4. Using the prepared pesto, toss the boiled zucchini noodles until well-covered.

5. If preferred, top the hot dish with cherry tomatoes.

Ready Time: fifteen minutes

Components:

- One lemon, juiced and zest

- Two tbsp of olive oil

- Four fish fillets

- Two tablespoons finely chopped fresh dill

- Flavor with salt and pepper

- Cut lemon slices to serve

Guidelines:

1. Turn the oven on to 375F, or 190C. Grease a baking plate with little olive oil.

2. Place the fish fillets in the ready baking plate. Olive oil should be sprinkled atop the plate, then salt,

pepper, lemon zest, and lemon juice should be sprinkled over it.

3. Scorch the cod fillets for 15 to 20 minutes in an oven that is already heated, or until the fish flake readily with a fork and is nontransparent.

4. For a zesty taste explosion, serve hot with lemon slices atop.

Set Up Time: fifteen minutes

Beef and Vegetables Kebabs:

Components:

- 1 pound (450g) of cubed, lean beef sirloin

- One bell pepper, sliced into pieces

- One red onion, chopped into pieces

- Eight small tomatoes

- Two teaspoons of olive oil

- 2 mashed garlic cloves

- One tsp of oregano, dried

- Flavor with salt and pepper

- Soak wooden skewers in water for half an hour

Guidelines:

1. To prepare a marinade, add olive oil, dried oregano, minced garlic, salt, and pepper in a basin.

2. Thread the beef cubes, cherry tomatoes, bell pepper, and red onion chunks, and substitute between the components onto the moistened wooden skewers.

3. After making the kebabs, move them to a shallow plate and overlay them with marinade, ensuring that they are coated completely. Cover it

and cool it for a minimum of 30 minutes.

4. Raise the grill's temp to medium-high. Turn the kebabs once or twice while grilling them for 8 to 10 minutes, or until the vegetables are tender and the beef is cooked to your preferred doneness.

5. Present hot, either by a fresh green salad or a side of steamed vegetables.

Set Aside Time: 45 min

Eggplant Lasagna:

Components:

- One large eggplant, cut lengthwise into thin slices

- Two cups marinara sauce (choose a reduced-sugar kind)

- One cup of ground mozzarella cheese

- One cup of low-fat cottage cheese

– A quarter cup of Parmesan cheese, grated

- One teaspoon of oregano, dried

One teaspoon of dried basil; salt and pepper to taste; optional garnish of fresh basil leaves

Guidelines:

1. Turn the oven on to 375F, or 190C. Lubricate a baking plate with a little quantity of olive oil.

2. Line the underside of the baking plate that has been prepared with a layer of eggplant slices. Drizzle the eggplant pieces with marinara sauce.

3. Put the low-fat cottage cheese, ground Parmesan and mozzarella

cheeses, dried basil, dried oregano, salt, and pepper in a saucer.

4. Overlay the marinara sauce with a layer of the cheese blend. Carry on with the layering until all components have been used, and then top with a film of cheese.

5. Simmer the baking plate for 30 minutes in a preheated oven overlaid with aluminum foil. After removing the foil, bake the cheese for a further 10 to 15 minutes, or until it is boiling and browned.

6. Prior to slicing, cool the lasagna for a few minutes. If preferred, garnish with fresh basil leaves just before serving.

Set Up Time: Half an hour

These tasty and nourishing Cruise Phase meals provide an excellent method to continue working toward your Dukan Diet weight loss objectives while savoring a variety of foods. Savor these tasty dishes as you move on to the next chapter of your culinary adventure!

Chapter Four

Consolidation Phase Recipes

The Consolidation Phase, which occurs as you move through the Dukan Diet, is an important time to sustain your weight loss while progressively adding a wider range of foods back into your diet. Lean proteins and non-starchy veggies will remain your top priorities throughout this phase, and you'll introduce other food groups in moderation. These recipes for the Consolidation Phase are made to promote your long-term success and well-being by providing you with tasty and satisfying meals as you move through this phase of your journey.

Quinoa Salad With Chicken:

Components:

- One cup of boiled quinoa

- One diced grilled chicken breast

- One cup of halved cherry tomatoes

- One diced cucumber

- A quarter cup of freshly sliced parsley

- A quarter cup of freshly sliced mint

- One tbsp of lemon juice

- Two tsp of olive oil

- Flavor with salt and pepper

- Garnish with crumbled feta cheese (optional)

Guidelines:

1. Put boiled quinoa, diced grilled chicken breast, sliced cucumber, split cherry tomatoes, chopped fresh parsley, and chopped fresh mint in a large saucer.

2. Mix olive oil, lemon juice, salt, and pepper in a small plate for the dressing.

3. Sprinkle the quinoa salad with the dressing and toss to coat uniformly.

4. If required, decorate with crumbled feta cheese prior to serving.

Set Up Time: fifteen minutes

Components:

Four bell peppers (deseeded)

- One cup of cooked brown rice

- One pound (450 grams) lean grated turkey

- One sliced onion

- Two crushed garlic cloves

- A single cup of tomato sauce

- 1 teaspoon each of dried oregano and basil

- Salt and pepper to relish

- Ground Parmesan cheese for decoration

Guidelines:

1. Set the oven to a temp of 375F, or 190C. Lubricate a baking dish with a little quantity of olive oil.

2. Cook the diced onion, minced garlic, and lean ground turkey in a frying pan using medium temp. until the onion becomes soft and the turkey is browned.

3. Fill the frying pan with the cooked brown rice, tomato sauce, dried basil, dried oregano, and salt and pepper. After mixing, heat for additional two to three minutes.

4. Softly press down to cram the packing into the bell peppers after filling them with the turkey and rice combination.

5. Move the packed bell peppers to the ready baking plate and overlay it with aluminum foil.

6. Scorch the bell peppers in the preheated oven for about half an hour, or until they are tender.

7. Remove the foil and overlay the stuffed bell peppers with ground Parmesan cheese. Return to the oven and scorch for a further five minutes, or until the cheese is foaming and thawed.

Set Up Time: 45 min

Ratatouille:

Components:

- 1 sliced eggplant

- 2 minced zucchini

- 2 diced yellow bell pepper

- 1 chopped red bell pepper

- 1 sliced onion

- 2 mashed garlic cloves

- 2 cups of sauced tomatoes

- Sliced fresh parsley to decorate

- Salt and pepper to taste

- One tsp each of dried thyme and dried basil

Guidelines:

1. In a large frying pan or Dutch oven, heat up the olive oil using medium temp. Put the diced onion, diced red bell pepper, diced yellow bell pepper, diced zucchini, diced eggplant, and minced garlic into the frying pan. Sauté the veggies, whisking occasionally, until they become tender.

2. Add tomato sauce, salt, pepper, dried basil, and dry thyme. Once

flavors are thoroughly combined, simmer, covered, whisking regularly, for 20 to 25 minutes.

3. Dress with nicely sliced fresh parsley and serve hot.

Set Up Time: thirty minutes

Lentil Soup:

Components:

- 1 cup of washed green lentils

- 1 sliced onion

- 2 sliced carrots

- 2 diced celery stalks

- 2 mashed garlic cloves

- Six cups of vegetable broth

- 1 teaspoon each of dried thyme and rosemary

- Flavor with salt and pepper

- Decorate with nicely sliced fresh parsley

Guidelines:

1. Mix the green lentils, vegetable broth, mashed garlic, dried thyme, dried rosemary, sliced onion, grated carrots, sliced celery, and salt and pepper in a large pan.

2. Allow the soup to boil using high temp. Then, reduce the temp to a simmer and cover the pot. Boil gently for 30 to 40 minutes, or until the veggies and lentils are soft.

3. Use salt and pepper to flavor. For a thicker consistency, you can partially mix the soup with an immersion blender, if you'd like.

4. Dress with freshly cut parsley and serve hot.

Set Up Time: Half an hour

Components:

- Two teaspoons olive oil

- Four beef sirloin steaks

- Two mashed garlic cloves

- 8 oz (225g) chopped mushrooms

- A quarter cup of Greek yogurt

- One cup of beef broth

- Flavor with salt and pepper

- Garnish with finely sliced fresh parsley

Guidelines:

1. Turn the heat up to medium-high on the grill. Add salt and pepper to the beef sirloin steaks for seasoning.

2. Cook the steaks on the grill for 4–5 minutes on each side, or until the preferred doneness is achieved. Remove the grill and give it a few minutes to rest.

3. In the meantime, bring a skillet's oil to a medium boil. Sliced mushrooms and minced garlic should be added to the skillet and cooked until the mushrooms are tender.

4. Add the Greek yogurt and beef stock, then boil the mixture for five to seven minutes, or until the sauce thickens.

5. Top the cooked steaks with a spoonful of mushroom sauce and fresh parsley that has been chopped.

Set Up Time: half an hour

These Consolidation Phase recipes provide you with a tasty and diverse range of dishes to enjoy as you continue your Dukan Diet journey toward sustaining your weight reduction and enhancing your general health. Savor each meal as it comes, and embrace the variety of flavors and healthy ingredients!

Chapter Five

Stabilization Phase Recipes

Congratulations on reaching the Dukan Diet's stabilization phase! This is the last part of your weight loss journey, during which you will concentrate on keeping the weight you have lost while indulging in a greater range of meals in moderation.

Balance, portion control, and sustainable lifestyle practices are prioritized during the stabilization phase to promote long-term weight management and general well-being. These recipes for the Stabilization Phase are meant to support you in continuing to lead a healthy lifestyle while enjoying delectable and filling meals.

Grilled Salmon With Asparagus and Lemon-Herb Butter:

Components:

- Four fillets of salmon

- One pound (450g) of trimmed asparagus spears

- Four tablespoons of softened unsalted butter

- 1 lemon's juice and zest

- 2 tbsp of freshly sliced parsley

- 1 tsp of freshly chopped dill

To taste, add salt and pepper.

Guidelines:

1. Set the grill's temperature to medium-high. Express lemon juice on top of the salmon fillets and spice with salt and pepper.

2. Cook the salmon fillets through and let it be flaky after grilling for 4–5 minutes on each side.

3. As you wait, blanch the asparagus spears for two to three minutes in steaming water, then empty out and pat dry.

4. A lemon-herb butter is made by mixing melted butter, lemon zest,

lemon juice, sliced fresh parsley, sliced fresh dill, salt, and pepper in a small saucer.

5. Top the grilled salmon with a dollop of lemon-herb butter and blanched asparagus spears and serve.

Twenty minutes for preparation

Quinoa-Stuffed Bell Peppers:

Components:

Four bell peppers, cut in half, and deseeded

One cup of cooked quinoa

One pound (450g) of grated chicken or turkey

One chopped onion and two minced garlic cloves

One cup of marinara sauce

One tsp of dehydrated oregano

One tsp of dried basil

To taste, add salt and pepper.

Parmesan cheese, ground, as a garnish

Guidelines:

1. Turn the oven on to 375F, or 190C. Lubricate a baking plate with a small quantity of olive oil.

2. Ground turkey or chicken, sliced onion, and mashed garlic should all be cooked in a frying pan using medium temperature until the meat is browned and the onion is soft.

3. Add the marinara sauce, salt, pepper, dried basil, dried oregano, and boiled quinoa. Boil gently for another two to three minutes.

4. Softly press down to squeeze the contents of the quinoa and meat combination into the halved bell peppers.

5. Cram the baking plate with the packed bell peppers. Bake for 25 to 30 minutes in a preheated oven with an aluminum foil cover.

6. After removing the foil, top the packed bell peppers with ground Parmesan cheese. Go back to the oven and bake for another five minutes, or until the cheese is bubbling and melted.

45 minutes for preparation

Greek salad With Grilled Chicken:

Components:

- Four cups of mixed salad greens and two grilled chicken breasts, chopped

- A quarter cup of crumbled feta cheese, minced one cup of - cherry tomatoes, halved 1/2 cup Kalamata olives, and 1 cucumber

- Two tbsp of pure olive oil

- One tbsp of vinegar made from red wine

- One tsp of dehydrated oregano

- To taste, add salt and pepper.

Guidelines:

1. Assorted salad greens, diced cucumber, split cherry tomatoes, pitted Kalamata olives, and crumbled feta cheese should all be mixed in a big saucer.

2. Combine the red wine vinegar, dried oregano, extra virgin olive oil, salt, and pepper in a tiny saucer to make a sauce.

3. Atop the salad, drizzle with the sauce and toss to coat uniformly.

4. After dividing the salad among dishes, place minced grilled chicken breasts over them.

5. If preferred, top with an additional drizzle of crumbled feta cheese and serve right away.

15 minutes for preparation

Vegetable Stir-Fry with Tofu:

Components:

14 oz (400g) extra-firm tofu, drained and pressed

2 tablespoons soy sauce (or tamari for a gluten-free option)

1 tablespoon rice vinegar

1 teaspoon sesame oil

1 tablespoon olive oil

2 mashed cloves of garlic

1 tbsp ground ginger

1 bell pepper, finely chopped

1 cup of broccoli florets

1 cup of minced mushrooms

Salt and pepper to relish

Sliced green onions for decoration

Guidelines:

1. Cut the pressed tofu into tiny cubes.

2. Inside a tiny saucer, beat together soy sauce, rice vinegar, and sesame oil to constitute a sauce.

3. Warm olive oil in a big frying pan or wok using medium-high temperature. Add mashed garlic and ground ginger, and cook for 1 minute until fragrant.

4. Introduce the tofu cubes into the frying pan and cook until all sides are golden brown, about 5-7 minutes.

5. Por the chopped bell pepper, broccoli florets, and sliced mushrooms to the frying pan, and cook for an extra 5 minutes or until vegetables are soft.

6. Spoon the sauce atop the tofu and vegetables, and toss to coat uniformly. Cook for a further 2-3 minutes until heated through.

Spice with salt and pepper to relish, and dress with sliced green onions before serving.

Prep Time: 30 minutes

Cauliflower Fried Rice:

Components:

- 1 head of cauliflower, ground or prepared such that it resembles rice

- Two tsp olive oil

- Two mashed garlic cloves

- One onion, two sliced carrots, one cup of frozen peas, two thawed eggs, three tsp of beaten soy sauce (or tamari for a gluten-free option), and one sliced onion

- 2 green onions cut thinly

To taste, add salt and pepper.

Guidelines:

1. In a large frying pan or wok, warm up the olive oil using medium temperature. Cook the sliced onion and mashed garlic until they become soft.

2. Cook the minced carrots in the frying pan for three to four minutes, or until they start to soften.

3. After shoving the veggies to one side of the frying pan, fill the vacant area with the beaten eggs. When the eggs are wholly cooked, scramble them and mix them with the vegetables.

4. When the cauliflower is tender, add the ground cauliflower to the frying

pan and boil gently, stirring regularly, for five to six minutes.

5. Add the soy sauce and thawed peas, then boil gently for another two to three minutes.

6. Before serving, add a dash of pepper and salt to flavor, and top with finely chopped green onions.

Twenty-five minutes for preparation

These recipes for the Stabilization Phase provide a diversity of tasty and nourishing options that will help realize your weight while still enjoying mouthwatering meals. Savor every meal as you proceed on your path to a better living by adopting a balanced eating pattern!

Tips for Success

Success with the Dukan Diet takes commitment to good living choices, consistency, and devotion. The following tips will help you make the most of the different diet phases and improve the chance that you will achieve your weight loss objectives:

1. Drink plenty of water: In addition to being helpful for general health, having lots of water can help handle wants and hunger. Try to have at least 8 glasses of water each day, and for variety, try adding plant teas and sweetened water.

2. Plan Your Meals: As food choices are more limited during the Attack and Cruise Phases, make the effort to plan your meals and snacks in advance. When hunger hits, making a plan ahead of time might help you avoid straying from your path and choosing dangerous foods.

3. Pay Attention to Lean Proteins: The Dukan Diet's cornerstone, lean

proteins, ought to be the focus of every meal. Select protein-rich foods such as low-fat dairy, lean meat, chicken, fish, and tofu to make sure you're getting enough to support muscle growth and repair.

4. Include Non-Starchy Vegetables: Vegetables that are not starchy are high in fiber, vitamins, and minerals, and they can help you feel satisfied and full all day. To add taste, color, and energy to your meals, include a range of bright veggies.

5. Limit Consuming Processed Foods: Steer clear of processed foods, sugary snacks, and high-fat foods as these can damage your attempts to lose weight. Rather, focus on eating full, nutrient-dense foods that will support your general health and feed your body.

6. Use serving Control Techniques: Even when eating Dukan-approved meals, pay attention to serving sizes and keep from overindulging. Serving yourself meals and snacks should involve using smaller bowls and plates and paying attention to amount sizes.

7. Pay Attention to Your Body: Be aware of your body's signs of hunger and fullness, and only eat when you are truly hungry. To truly enjoy every bite, practice careful eating and learn to distinguish between cravings that are driven by mood or boredom and bodily hunger.

8. Include Physical Exercise: Any weight loss program should include regular physical exercise since it can

improve metabolism, burn calories, and boost general health. Choose fun hobbies and try to get in at least 30 minutes of exercise each day of the week.

9. Exercise Perseverance and Patience: Being patient and persistent is crucial when trying to lose weight since it takes time, especially when you hit plateaus or experience poor progress. Have faith in the process, keep your focus on your objectives, and acknowledge and value your growth.

10. Ask for Help: Be in the company of friends, family, or other Dukan Diet adherents who can provide duty, drive, and support. Talk to people about your successes and problems, and don't be afraid to ask for help or support when you need it.

Your weight loss goals and the enjoyment of a better, happy lifestyle are within reach if you stick to the Dukan Diet's rules and utilize these helpful ideas. Recall that making long-lasting changes that support long-term health and well-being is what describes success rather than simply hitting a certain number on the scale.

Meal Planning and Preparation

To be successful on the Dukan Diet, you need to carefully plan and prepare your meals. Ensure you always have healthy options available and prevent yourself from looking for bad options when you're hungry by taking the effort to plan your meals earlier and prepare good foods. The following tips will assist you in planning and making Dukan meals:

1. Allocate Time for Planning: Set out time every week to prepare your meals for the next days. This could happen on a Saturday afternoon or at any other time that is suitable for you. Setting out a certain time for planning will keep you focused and organized as you work toward your eating goals.

2. Make a Weekly Menu: Write down a list of the foods you'll be eating that week, or use a meal planner. Consider your dietary needs, plan, and any important events or times that might affect the meals you choose. At every meal, try to strike a mix between non-starchy veggies, lean proteins, and healthy fats.

3. Consciously Purchase: After you've planned your meals, continue to the

grocery store with a buying list of the items you'll need. Steer clear of the areas holding processed and high-calorie meals and stay around the store's edges, which is where the fresh fruit, lean proteins, and dairy products are found.

4. Batch Cooking: Think about making some of your meals ahead of time, including cooked grains, roasted veggies, or grilled chicken. You may save time during the week and ease the process of putting together healthy meals when you're pressed for time by prepping these things beforehand.

5. Assemble Ingredients in Advance: When you return from the shopping store, spend some time preparing the things. So that your meats are set to cook when you need them, wash and chop your veggies, portion out your

snacks, and prepare them. To keep cooked things fresh, store them in the refrigerator in sealed cases.

6. Invest in Time-Saving Tools: If you're looking to speed up the meal preparation process, think about getting cooking tools like a food processor, Instant Pot, or slow cooker. Using these tools will enable you to make meals more quickly and with less effort.

7. Make a Leftovers Plan: Accept leftovers as an easy method to eat healthy meals without having to prepare them from scratch every single day. Make extra food and put the leftovers in different containers so you can quickly reheat it for lunches or dinners during the week.

8. Show Flexibility: Meal preparation is vital, but when life finally throws curveballs, it's also critical to be changeable and flexible. If your plans change or you don't follow your meal plan exactly, don't worry. Keep your attention on picking the best course of action for you in each case and don't let mistakes hold you back.

9. Test Out Some New Recipes: Try out different recipes and taste combinations to make mealtimes interesting and fascinating. To keep your meals delicious and filling, try with different herbs, spices, and cooking techniques.

10. Remain Organized: To make meal preparation easy, keep your kitchen well-stocked with necessary supplies and equipment. To reduce clutter and keep your office organized, set aside

specific places for the keeping of culinary tools, fresh veggies, and pantry basics. Then, clean up as you go.

You'll position yourself for success on the Dukan Diet and create a lasting and pleasurable lifestyle by heeding these guidelines and putting meal planning and preparation into your daily routine. Keep in mind that persistence is important and that making tiny, manageable changes over time might result in significant advancements toward your wellbeing and health goals.

Grocery Shopping Tips

A vital part of the Dukan Diet is food shopping since the meals you bring into your home have an instant effect on your ability to follow the plan and reach your weight loss goals. The following tips will help you shop at the food store and make good decisions:

1. Make a List: Make a list of the things you need and take stock of what you already have at home before you go to the food shop. To make sure you don't forget anything, order your list according to food groups (such as dairy, veggies, and meats).

2. Adhere to the Boundaries: Fresh veggies, lean meats, and dairy items are usually found along the store's perimeter in most grocery shops. The bulk of Dukan-approved foods are found in these outer areas, so focus your shopping efforts there.

3. Select Whole Foods: Whenever possible, choose whole, lightly cooked foods. Select lean meat, chicken, fish, eggs, and low-fat dairy items over pre-packaged or cooked foods. Also, consider fresh fruits and veggies.

4. Carefully Read Labels: Spend some time reading the labels, studying the ingredients list, and checking the nutrition information when picking packaged foods. Seek things with low amounts of dangerous fats, sodium, and added sugars. Steer clear of goods with long lists of fake additives and preservatives.

5. Give Lean Proteins Priority: The Dukan Diet is based mostly on lean proteins, so make sure to stock up on a range of protein sources, including low-fat dairy products, fish, tofu,

eggs, and chicken breast. Before cooking, pick lean meat cuts and remove any obvious fat.

6. Consume More Vegetables: A sizable percentage of your meals should consist of non-starchy veggies, which are an important component of the Dukan Diet. Pick a range of bright veggies to add taste, texture, and nutrients to your meals, such as spinach, bell peppers, broccoli, cauliflower, and leafy greens.

7. Add Nutritious Fats: Although the Dukan Diet has a strong focus on lean meats, it's also critical to include healthy fats in your diet for general health and pleasure. Select foods like avocado, nuts, seeds, olive oil, and fatty fish like mackerel and salmon that are rich in healthy fats.

8. Pick Up Essentials: Stock your kitchen with whole grains (quinoa, brown rice), legumes (chickpeas, lentils), herbs, spices, and low-sodium broths or stocks—essential staples that are in keeping with the Dukan Diet rules.

9. Limit Consuming Processed Foods: Avoid processed foods, sugary snacks, and high-calorie sweets as these can interfere with your Dukan Diet success making it impossible for you to shed fats and develop muscles as an athlete. Aim to fill your cart with entire, nutrient-dense foods rather than sweets like chips, cookies, candies, and other tempting aisles.

10. Shop Mindfully: Avoid rash purchases by taking your time and

making careful choices. Don't shop while you're hungry, follow your list, and pay attention to the amounts and serve sizes. Shopping during off-peak hours can help you escape crowds and lessen your temptation.

You can make healthier eating a long-term part of your lifestyle and stay on track with the Dukan Diet by using these food shopping ideas and making smart decisions at the store. With every grocery shop visit, keep in mind to favor nutrient-dense foods, make a plan, and maintain your attention on your general wellness and health goals.

Eating Out on the Dukan Diet

You don't have to lose progress while on the Dukan Diet if you eat out. You can relish eating out without sacrificing your health and weight loss objectives if you prepare ahead of time and exercise attentiveness. If you choose to eat out on the Dukan Diet, the following advice will help you navigate restaurants and choose healthier options:

1. Check Out Menus Ahead: Nowadays, a lot of restaurants have their menus available online, which makes it easier to browse selections and schedule your lunch in advance. Before you go, examine the menu and point out items like salads, grilled proteins, and vegetable-based dishes that follow the Dukan Diet principles.

2. Select Meals Based on Protein: Seek for recipes that highlight lean proteins, such as fish, grilled chicken, or lean turkey or beef cuts. Steer clear of fried and breaded foods and instead

use grilling, broiling, or steaming techniques.

3. Request Modifications: Never be embarrassed to ask for dietary adjustments from your server. Ask for dressing on the side, ask for grilled or steamed veggies in place of fries or mashed potatoes, or request for a side salad in place of a starchier side dish.

4. Take Note of Portion Sizes: Be mindful of portion sizes at restaurants as they are usually greater than what you would eat at home. You might share an entree or ask for a to-go box to divide out half of your meal before you start eating.

5. Pay Attention to Non-Starchy Vegetables: Fill up on non-starchy veggies to give your dish more

substance and nutrition without consuming extra calories. Look for vegetable-based meals such as stir-fries or grilled vegetable platters, or salads and vegetable side dishes.

6. Maximum Additional Items: Sauces, garnishing, and condiments with a lot of added sugar, fat, or calories should be avoided. To restrict your consumption, request sauces on the side and use them sparingly. When feasible, go for basic dressings made with olive oil and vinegar or vinaigrettes.

7. Remain Hydrated: To assist you feel full and avoid overindulging, sip lots of water both before and throughout your meal. Water, unsweetened tea, or sparkling water with a squeeze of lime or lemon are better options than sugary drinks.

8. Use Portion Control Techniques: Observe serving sizes and refrain from overindulging in foods heavy in fat or calories. Rather than to stop eating when you are extremely full, try to enjoy your meal leisurely and relish every bite.

9. Exercise Flexibility: Request changes or substitutes if you can't find something on the menu that works for you. Don't be afraid to be inventive. Numerous eateries are open to meeting your nutritional requirements and can alter dishes to suit your preferences.

10. Appreciate the Experience: Keep in mind that having a meal out and interacting with loved ones is just as vital as the cuisine. Pay attention to

the company and the discussion rather than obsessing over maintaining a strict diet.

You can continue to make progress toward your health and weight loss objectives by adhering to the Dukan Diet for athletes and making wise decisions when dining out. You can prioritize your health and well-being and still enjoy dining out with a little preparation and mindfulness.

Staying Motivated

It might be tough to keep drive when following the Dukan Diet, or any diet, especially when you're going through different steps and running against roadblocks. But constant motivation is important to long-term success. Here are some tips to keep you inspired and committed to meeting your weight reduction and health objectives:

1. Establish Specific, Achievable Goals: Establish important, attainable goals that are specific for you. Having specific objectives keeps you motivated and offers you something to aim for, whether your goal is to improve your general health, fit into your best pair of pants, or lose a specific amount of weight.

2. Track Your growth: Regularly record your weight, measures, and other important data to keep tabs on your development. Gaining clear results over time will greatly inspire you and improve your desire to follow the Dukan Diet.

3. Celebrate Your wins: No matter how small your wins may be, recognize them. Celebrate your small wins along the road, no matter how big or small—like meeting a goal, avoiding temptation, or following your weekly eating plan.

4. Find Your Why: Consider the reasons you initially started on the Dukan Diet, and whenever you feel your commitment lessening, bring them to mind. Rediscovering your "why" can help you find your drive again, whether it's for health reasons, confidence building, or to set a good example for others.

5. Visualize Your Goals: Make a vision board or picture the achievement of your goals. Imagine your look and feelings when you hit other goals or reach your goal weight.

Especially in trying situations, visualizing your success can help you stay motivated and focused.

6. Remain Informed: Learn about the Dukan Diet and its driving ideas. Knowing the science of the diet and how it works can help you stay committed to your goals and give you the confidence to make decisions that will help you reach them.

7. Ask for Help: Assemble a network of friends, family, or Dukan Diet participants who are helpful and able to provide responsibility, motivation, and direction. Talk to people about your accomplishments and difficulties, and when things get hard, depend on your network of support.

8. Make Self-Compassion a Practice: Throughout your road, remember to treat yourself with love and self-compassion. Recognize that hurdles and setbacks are normal parts of the process, and try not to be too hard on yourself if things don't always go according to plan. Show yourself the same care and kindness that you would show a friend.

9. Remain Motivated: Look for inspiration in the form of success tales, inspiring sayings, or before-and-after pictures of people who have followed the Dukan Diet and achieved. Be in the company of happy people who push you to keep going forward.

10. Pay Attention to Non-Scale Wins: Keep in mind that following the Dukan Diet right means more than

just your weight. Acknowledge non-quantitative wins like heightened energy, better physical health, restful sleep, and improved general happiness as signs of progress and success.

You may keep your drive and attention on your health and weight loss goals while following the Dukan Diet by putting these methods into your daily practice. Though your motivation may change over time, you can beat hurdles and achieve long-term success by staying driven, reliable, and strong.

Conclusion

In summary, beginning the Dukan Diet is a step toward more wellbeing, improved health, and long-term weight loss. Numerous delectable and nutritious meals that support your goals for the complete diet have been discovered by you on this culinary adventure. You now know how to choose meals with awareness and purpose, embracing healthy fats, non-starchy veggies, and wholesome nutrition to fuel your body and uplift your spirit. All of the attack's phases have been addressed, along with the phases of consolidation, cruise, and stabilization.

Remember that success on the Dukan Diet is more about your sensible lifestyle choices and good habits than it is about the numbers on the scale when you reflect on your experiences. No matter what your fitness level is— be it reaching your target weight, stepping up the intensity of your workout, or simply learning more about portion sizes and nutrition— celebrate each victory as a step toward your optimum health.

After you've finished this cookbook, prioritize your health and well-being and make choices that are consistent with your goals and values. Never forget that you have a daily chance to take care of your body, mind, and spirit by maintaining a healthy diet, getting regular exercise, and engaging in self-care. Keep up your motivation and seek out community support.

We are appreciative of your decision to adhere to the Dukan Diet, a gourmet quest for vitality and health. I hope these recipes may inspire and brave you in the years to come as you adopt a wellness and well-being lifestyle. I hope your trips are filled with happiness and good fortune! Salutations!